America On The Couch

Dr. Richard Waldron

Being Worthy LLC

CONTENTS

Chapter One

Not Feeling Well? Maybe It's Not You. It's All Of Us

My name is Richard Walrdon and I am a Psychologist and Psychiatric Nurse Practitioner. I have been providing mental health treatment for over 35 years and I keep hearing the same thing from the people I'm working with in session.

"I think it's me. Sometimes I think that I'm making this stuff up. You know, like it's all in my head and I'm trying to figure it out."'

"Like what the fuck is going on?!"

"I just feel so keyed up. Edgy. And then so really down and depressed like I can't get out of my own way."

"There's really no good news and nobody seems to care or give a shit. It keeps me up at night. Then I'm on social media or doom scrolling and I feel worse.

The next day, I'm tired and dragging my ass around. I think I need to go on Prozac or something."

Well, maybe it's not you. Would you consider for a moment that it's not you at all?

On an average year, I will perform nearly two thousand hours of talk therapy and write hundreds of prescriptions for people who really benefit from them. What's nice is to see people get better from the work we do.

Fear, anxiety, depression, insomnia and negativity seem to be all around us.

For many, it causes hopelessness, powerlessness and emotional paralysis. People feel that they have little control over much of what happens in their lives and they become desperate for answers. Just getting accurate information is a problem. Just when we think we know something, we doubt what we read, hear or see.

This is all happening as artificial intelligence is becoming part of our lives and a fact of life, like it or not.

So, I have come to the monumental realization that so many of the issues that people present to me are not just in their head.

What if you are, in fact, having a normal reaction to an abnormal situation?

You're not crazy. The larger societal situation is creating hatred, fear, division and doubt in everything you know and feel?

Instead of you being on my couch, I think it's time for Uncle Sam and Lady Liberty to spend some time getting their gyros reset.

America on the Couch is a book that will help you gain perspective and help you see how the forces of American life are making us physically, financially, spiritually and emotionally ill.

You are just responding normally to what's going on.

Chapter Two

Uncle Sam And Lady Liberty... Let's Just Say That They Have Some Issues

Let's pretend for a moment that Uncle Sam and Lady Liberty made an appointment with me to come in for some couples therapy.

Neither of them are particularly happy. In fact, Lady Liberty is seriously thinking about going back to France.

Dr. Rich: Good Morning. It's good to see you both. Please have a seat on the couch.

Lady Liberty: If it's ok with you, I'm going to put the torch down over here... oui. Bonjour, comment ça? Bien non? I'm practicing my French. I may be going back to Paris. Ever since Sam got a stupid cell phone he can't get off of it. Right, Sam? Sam? Sam!!

Uncle Sam: What? Oui. Whatever you say Libby.

Libby: I used to be up on a pedestal and admired by all, especially Sam.   Now I can't get anyone's attention.

Sam: I just have to finish this parlay. And there, done!

Libby: The only parlay I know is parlez, which means talk in French. Speak to me Sam!

Dr.Rich: How long have you two had trouble talking to each other?

Libby: Maybe 10 years? Dix ans...

Sam: I didn't know we had a problem, doc. Really. I was just doin' what everyone else does.

Libby: I just feel all alone. Like I'm on an island while everything is going on around me. Nothing good. People in America are unhappy. They just don't care about how Sam and I put this all together, and it seems like it's all coming apart.

Sam: I really like this cell phone. It's got all those cool apps. I have 335 million followers! Libby, I can be an influencer!

Libby: You've been an influencer since 1776,.... without that thing! I swear, Doc, he's on that thing 24 hours a day.

Sam: Aw. Not that much. Let me check my usage. Oh it's a lot. Only 18 hours.

Libby: All your waking hours!!

Sam: Yeah, you're right. I'm not getting much sleep. I'm always tired. Hey Doc, you got something for that? Maybe some Adderall?

Dr. Rich: No Adderall Sam. It seems like you compulsively use that phone and are distracted.

Sam: Maybe...?!

Libby: I tried telling him that they're trying to get rid of all the people who came here for a better life. I got a poem by my feet. You may know it, Doc.

Those aren't just words. It's what America is about, but these days it's yada-yada-yada.

Sam: What people don't realize is, except for the Lenape and other indigenous people, everyone came from somewhere else.

Libby: Even me. I came over on an old boat. The trip across the Atlantic was rough. I was in pieces...

Sam: When she got here, Libby watched millions get processed next door at Ellis Island. Once done, they headed out, not knowing what to expect, but the opportunity was there to live free and do better. And they did.

Libby: They forgot. And now they hate the “others”.

Sam: America is not a gated community.

Dr. Rich: Let's get back to why you’re here.

Libby: Sam is getting to be like everyone else here in America. He's distracted, he has stopped using his brain. You know, he's very wise and he's watching all these games, violent shows about murders, investigations, and zombies. I swear that if he buys an Xbox or Playstation, I'm gone. Adieu!

Sam: I don't want that, Doc. Thinking takes too much effort. I don't want to know, I just want to be happy. I'm confused and also so bored and nervous. Libby catches me just scrolling…

Dr.Rich: That's called doom scrolling.

Sam: I'm just so down and don't know what to do anymore. Just so stuck.

Dr.Rich: Well, you can get unstuck if you stop doing what you are doing Sam and maybe show others in America that they can too.

Libby: You have to believe in what we stood for together. You know, grow a set. Put down the phone. Look up. Go outside. America, the beautiful. We had our people die for us and others are dying to be here.

Sam: I'm worried about our little ones. They need to know how we got here. Our story. It's a great one. We've made many mistakes and things aren't great now, but we eventually got it right.

Dr. Rich: Sam and Libby, let me ask you something. Are we worthy of you? The sacrifices you made, the values you hold dear?

Libby: I was beginning to think, non! I'm going back. A lot of Americans want to leave and go elsewhere. But sitting here, I'm thinking now, we've got to teach the people that democracy needs to be fought for every day. I'm fighting, Sam, for us, in this session!

Sam: The people are worthy of us, Libby. We have to get them to care. To wake up. To demand justice, accountability and build rather than destroy. They are basically good people who were purposely distracted so that bad leaders could do what they wanted for themselves.

Libby: It doesn't work that way. I'm pretty pissed off. I just realized that!

Dr Rich: What's making you angry?

Libby: That Americans allowed this to happen! They believe what they want to believe and are so easily misled, fed a fire hose of garbage to become overwhelmed and then tune out.

Sam: Look at me. I'm an example.

Libby: What I really can't stand is when half of America stays home and doesn't vote. It's too cold. It's too hot. It's too far. It doesn't make a difference.

Dr.Rich: That's how people got to feeling powerless.

Sam: I love Libby. Especially when she gets fired up. *Je' taime, ma chere!* I have to get off my butt and stop this stupid distraction. I didn't realize how politics, money and the media grabbed the power away from us. I fell asleep on the job.

Libby: We've got a lot of work to do, thanks Doc. I have one last question. How do we pay for this session?

Dr. Rich: You have Medicare and a good supplement that will pay me 96%. We're good. See you next time.

Sam: Everybody should have this. Let's go Libby!

Chapter Three

How COVID-19 Radically Changed American Life

In a mental health practice, most people who seek out help have an intolerable degree of anxiety and depression. It is staggering to me to learn how many experienced the onset of their symptoms just as the COVID-19 pandemic began to subside.

When the "world opened up again", something we all longed for during our extra space mandated quarantine, the collective post traumatic stress emerged in full force. There is a weird amnesia pervasive in our culture regarding the pandemic. People seemingly want to forget wearing masks, staying indoors and being in front of a computer screen-if they had a computer.

America lost 1.1 million people due to COVID-19. It is estimated that vaccines saved more than 3 million. Initially, we were horrified to learn that 2,500 people died. Then, it grew into the thousands and hundreds of thousands lost. To put it into context, the US lost the population of Rhode Island. Everybody knows someone who died of COVID-19.

We don't like to think about the enormity of this pandemic. Do we tolerate death more now?

But when I take a view of history, I do ask how people dealt with COVID-19. Are they still dealing with it (long COVID) and are their psychiatric symptoms correlated to that time?

My observation is that COVID-19 has profoundly changed our individual patterns of behavior, and collectively how we view our lives and each other.

What became abnormal, in many ways, remains abnormal without knowing what a new normal would look like.

First, the positives:

We are looking at how we work differently. Much has been said about work/life balance. Working at home, if possible, provided greater autonomy, flexibility and time to do other things other than commuting. People resigned from unworthy jobs.

It gave rise to telehealth which made physical and emotional care efficiently delivered, particularly in rural areas. More online courses became accessible to those who wanted to further their education. If people had money, time, a computer, internet service, and cell phone access, transmission, speed became faster.

The delivery services such as DoorDash and Amazon flourished as did UPS, Fedex, and the USPS. We drove less, which helped the environment and temporarily lowered the energy costs.

People learned about FaceTime. What would have happened to all of us if we couldn't see those we loved and cared about?

We learned how critically important our first responders are, many of whom died in the pandemic. Similarly, thousands of health care workers died giving life saving treatment to those who came down with the virus.

COVID-19 led to the discovery of using mRNA to begin degrading the replication of the virus. By tweaking a vaccine for the SARS virus, it was possible to deliver a vaccine for COVID-19 and treatment, when detected early that proved effective.

Finally, we are more aware of the fragility of our mental health and are talking about it more. People are more apt to seek out treatment.

How have we changed?

We don't gather at homes as much as we did in the prior decades. Social distancing in the long term has reduced the frequency of home visits and dinner parties. Do you find you don't hug as much? Many people are less touchy-feely.

The pandemic forced people to be isolated. This has led to loneliness on a large scale, particularly among the elderly. The resulting depression has led to increases in addiction and suicide rates. Do you find yourself more withdrawn and disconnected? Less motivated to seek the company of others?

How are you sleeping? Many people are not sleeping well due to too many negative thoughts at night, being keyed up and on edge. They worry about everything. Will I have a job? Will I be able to pay my bills? Will I have health insurance and other existential, anxiety-producing matters. Nothing is taken for granted.

We are losing faith in getting accurate information from our leaders and our institutions.

How did this happen?

The COVID-19 pandemic occurred because of a failure of imagination and preparation. Without any experience with anything of such magnitude, the pillars of our society were operating in a fog of war without clear understanding and facts. Those responsible were left guessing about effective courses of action.

When people panicked and wanted to know what to do, the last thing they wanted to hear was "I don't know". "I don't know" leads to official statements like "we're looking at this strongly and have it under control. We'll be coming out with a statement shortly".

Remember that in the initial months of the COVID-19 pandemic, there was no effective treatment. So public health officials were left with a horrifying reality. America needed to isolate, quarantine and shut down to prevent contagion and more wide scale death.

What also occurred was denial, minimization and grossly contradictory information as the illness and death toll mounted. Why is this happening? Who do we hold accountable? We need someone to blame.

And the blame came. COVID-19 gave rise to all kinds of conspiracy theories that exist today and shape our politics, public policy and community health agendas.

In the absence of a unified statement, people went into their media silos and social media to hear what they thought they needed to hear or wanted to hear.

To mask or not to mask. That was the question. And if your opinion was different, things became hostile, depending upon where you stood on the political spectrum. At times, it became violent, egged on by media coverage.

And so, the distrust has proliferated and has turned personal with negative regard for anything authoritative. There's almost a perverse pleasure in a win-lose culture. "Owning the Libs, shutting up the stupid MAGA's"-everyone loses and nothing constructive changes.

If someone wears a mask today on a flight, other passengers may give the evil, side-eye disapproving glance. Perhaps that individual has respiratory issues like COPD and real immense fears about getting ill. Perhaps that person is following health care providers preventative instructions.

The COVID-19 pandemic has changed the way people under 25 meet, speak, socialize and date. Educators and mental health providers noted that from 2020 onward, teenagers became used to being on screens. They don't pick up in-person social cues very well, may not put the effort into the healthy vanity of cleaning up for others and would rather stay in their bedrooms than go outside.

For many college students, it may be their first time dating. Many do not know how to deal with conflicts in their new relationships or negotiate their initial sexual encounters. Accustomed to being on social media and saying anything they want, it is a very different interaction live, in real- time. The aggrieved content doesn't change and is normalized.

People are dating less and more unlikely to be in long-term committed relationships, to marry and have children. In time, our population could decrease with dire economic outcomes.

There's a general disgust with dating apps. Besides bars and alternative places to gather (dating at work is dangerous), where do you meet people? Worse, people often misrepresent themselves on profiles. When people give up trying to partner up, this inevitably creates futility, pessimism, depression, isolation and despair.

Nurses and physicians died during the pandemic. Some died by suicide, not being able to cope with so much disease, lack of ventilators or treatment and patients constantly dying. They were forced into

18-24 hour shifts that led to increased exposure and their own deaths as well.

While there is an excellent career market in health care, not enough students are entering the field due to the cost of education, years needed to become proficient and not having control of their work flow.

Nurses are burning out and are leaving the profession at alarming rates. There has been a nursing shortage since the beginning of the century and remains today. The National Institute of Health, The Center for Disease Control and The Department of Health and Human Services have been gutted as some of the most brilliant researchers have been let go.

So, if this all sounds pretty miserable and crazy, guess what? It is and it's not normal! It's also external to you and you are reacting normally to these weird and irrational situations

We have to get smarter, not accept the status quo and not drive like Thelma and Lousie, off the proverbial cliff.

In later chapters, I'll challenge you to change the powerless way you think and fight for a healthier America.

To this day, there is no national memorial for the first responders and healthcare workers. care workers.

To this day, there is no national memorial for the 1,100,000 who perished from COVID-19.

Chapter Four

WHAT IF WE LIVED IN A COMMONWEALTH? WAIT, SOME OF US DO!

If you live in Virginia, Pennsylvania, Kentucky or Massachusetts, yours is both a state and a Commonwealth. Once you discover the philosophy of Commonwealth governance, you'd be very impressed. So much so, you would want everyone to enjoy the benefits of this form of political organization.

First, a lesson in political science and civics is necessary. A "Commonwealth" is a form of government that focuses on the common good. This means adhering to the rule of law, protection of individual rights, fostering community and shared responsibility. Historically, such entities shared ownership of resources, promoted cohesion toward a unified sense of well-being. If I did well, I would want you to do well and we will help you do so, if you needed.

William Penn founded the colony of Pennsylvania, which later became an aforementioned Commonwealth. Quakers were persecuted for their views of peaceful interactions, correcting social injustice of violence and equality in England. The Society of Friends brought to America the political ethics of collaboration, consensus building, and shared accountability,

Commonwealth, as a conceptual foundation of a given society, arose as a response to the promotion of basic worthiness and brotherly love. There are several functional principles upon which the Commonwealth is rooted.

1. **Public participation -** In order for a commonwealth to thrive, citizens must actively become involved in decision making. This leads to the formation and implementation of rational public policy to solve challenges. Every year, America has primaries and elections to vote for candidates. There are debates and live and/or electronic public forums to find consensus.

2. **Accountability and transparency** - In a commonwealth or a democracy, the public through

an informed independent media, holds leaders to a record of their service. Any potential corruption is exposed with the bad actor being expelled from their service in an America that cares.

3. **Sustainability and cooperation -** Just as in colonial times, the commonwealth philosophy promoted long term growth and survival of its citizenry

4. **Building community cohesion** -The commonwealth philosophy brings people together with unity even when options differ. It is fine to disagree and give voice to contrasting views as long as it's done in a dignified and respectful manner and not systematically silenced.

5. **Versatility and resilience** - A major advantage of commonwealth and its emphasis upon the common good is when we are faced with looming existential challenges. With it's flexible political structure, commonwealth or democracy can swiftly adept to large scale problems and quickly assure rebuilding.

6. **Commonwealths provided balance** -Fairness, justice and balance are critical values. We try to find equitable ways to improve the lives of less fortunate individuals. This promotes homeostatic stability within its citizenry and is a mainstay feature.

There are contrasting differences in a commonwealth that distinguish it compared to other political philosophies.

1. **Commonwealth versus Autocracy** - Autocracy centralizes political power and influence in one person or a small group, disregarding the common good and wider public interest. Commonwealths prioritize fairness and the rule of law to benefit the entire community. Autocracies exist for the benefit of those on top.

2. **Commonwealth versus Republic** -Republics emphasize individual rights and freedoms with less focus upon the collective whole.

3. **Commonwealth versus Socialism** - Capitalism thrives in a commonwealth where individuals can pursue or create resilient, self-sufficient economies. Socialism is all about the collective, regardless of whether the common good is met. The majority of a country's individual resources are gathered and redistributed.

4. **Commonwealth versus communism** -Communism emphasizes a total adherence to the state. All efforts and resources are given to the state. Everyone is on an equal footing no matter

their contribution. Individuality is denied. The state controls every aspect of life.

America was essentially an expression of the purest form of commonwealth. Now it is really a hybrid that borrows parts of different governance philosophies.

Now, hold on a minute! I think someone needs some therapy.....

If Uncle Sam were on my couch, I think I would be treating him for depression and anxiety. I think, part of the session would go like this:

Uncle Sam: Uh man... I really feel bad today. Soon, I'm going to be 250 and that's nice and what-not. But, people don't get me. I mean, I don't think they care about me.

Dr. Rich: Yeah, I can see that. Why do you think that people don't care?

Uncle Sam: I love all my people. I want them all to be well, you know? I want them to look out for each other. If they need a helping hand, I'm there for them. I don't understand why they all can't get along.

Dr. Rich: I'll bet it keeps you up at night worrying about them and what will be.

Uncle Sam: You got that right! We've always have had problems, but most of the time, we have smart, caring people to get us through the bad times. I don't see that now. I'm sorry. I have this awful headache...

Dr. Rich: You really are hurting these days and...

Uncle Sam: And the worst of it, is that I feel like I'm coming apart, Everybody is out for themselves. They are all on their cells doing all kinds of nonsense that gets them distracted. Including me.

Dr. Rich: You sound like they don't care if you matter or not.

Uncle Sam: Look, I fought to be here and I stood up for those who wanted to destroy me. Today, people have forgotten about that. When did my story become unimportant? They don't teach history and civics in school. There are a lot of people spreading rumors that just aren't there. The rich, they lie!!

Dr Rich: You were always strong because your people stood united.

Uncle Sam: I was telling Liberty the other day that we were once a beacon of hope. She's still standing with that torch. She said to me "Sam, don't get down. I still hold that light and maybe our people will look for it again. But I think you need some help and should talk to someone". And that's why I'm here. I don't want to say it but maybe I'm just an old man and my time has passed.

Dr. Rich: Sam, I'm writing this book called *America on the Couch*. Isn't it ironic that you're on my couch? I'm hoping it will turn things around. You're not the only one who's feeling bad, Sam. It's not that knowing that is going to help that much, but I'm trying to tell everyone that the reasons they feel nervous and sad is the same as yours. All the outside external stuff. They, like you, are reacting normally to an abnormal situation.

Uncle Sam: Yeah, that's right.

Dr. Rich: What, you're about Sam. What you believe in and what you've shown the world is right and good. The people have lost their way but they can find their way back if they agree to do it and hang together.

Uncle Sam: Yeah, do their part, make a difference. Do good things. Watch out for each other. Put down the bad stuff. Get rid of corrupt idiots. Help out others. Be kind and polite. Be respectful to our friendly countries. Fight the evil ones when we must.

Dr. Rich: You just need people to care and support all the good things you stand for.

Uncle Sam: If people did that, things would get better. They would feel and be better. And if they're better, I'll be better.

Dr Rich: You got this Sam.

Uncle Sam: We got this if we all get each other. By the way, your book sounds great. Good luck with it!

Chapter Five

How Ratings Make Us Discontent!

We can all agree that it's nice to feel content with your life. For many of us, that's not always possible and for others seemingly impossible. "I just want to be happy", is a phrase often said. The problem with that is happiness is nearly impossible to maintain. I equate that word with euphoria-feeling high, flying high.

Humans and all living organisms seek balance or homeostasis. When we are talking about this as it applies to our emotions, what we really want is to feel solid, stable and content. When we are upset, we struggle to get back to our baseline, to keep on an even keel. Once there, we desire contentment.

Another element towards feeling content is our personal sense of self-worth. I describe the fundamental cornerstone of our being as worthiness in *Being Worthy*. In my way of thinking, we are all born worthy and our individual experiences build upon that fundamental cornerstone or erode and destroy it.

Another of the many ways that our societal processes negatively impact our lives is our obsession with measurement, matrices and ratings.

How many times a day are you asked to rate people, places, services or things? How do you rate? And by the way, how to rank or rate yourself?

Alexa just decided to pop in and ask me to rate my recent purchase of lemon snap cookies.

Really? Seriously??

Why can't I just experience the pleasure of having a few cookies without considering how I actually feel about them?

And that's the problem.

Constant ratings are destroying our personal sense of contentment, always throwing us off in small and big ways. The subtleties of ratings are that it's never enough. We are pushed to want more or "help people to make better choices". Why can't we make these choices ourselves on our own without compiled data? Who is compiling the data and for what purpose (consumerism? profit?)?

Let's dive in, for a moment, to what you're doing when you rate. You are asked to evaluate and judge the worthiness and value of what you're rating along some continuum. This is usually along a line of what's "good" versus "bad". Ratings are therefore subjective; subject to the agenda and bias of those doing the judging. This has become so subconscious that we accept continuous rating and judgment as normal in our everyday lives.

In the words of Pink, "Why do we do that? Why do we do that? Why do we do that?!"

When ratings are applied to us continuously, we become fearful of judgment – particularly negative judgment. We begin to become defensive, fear-based and less confident. Over the course of time and in extreme, people become fearful of potential failure and inadequacy. One can feel that everything doesn't matter.

And there you have it. Anxiety, depression and despair.

Our media provides constant idealized images of what we should be, according to some consumer-driven standard. You are not enough unless you buy this product. Shrewd marketing creates unhealthy and unfair comparisons among people. It's compare and despair time, all the time, 24/7.

Within the psychology of compare and despair, made possible by matrices and rating, nobody can achieve contentment. There is envy and jealousy. "I want that and I can't have it. It's not fair!" Worse,"I'm not worthy because I suck. I don't deserve good things in my life".

Chronic fear of negative judgment ruins risk taking, initiative and creativity. People don't try out new hobbies or interests because they are not instantly proficient. "I always wanted to play guitar but I'm probably not going to be good at it." Yes, Dave Grohl would agree that when you first try to play, you're not going to sound good. If you suck at it eventually you'll get three chords down and play simple songs. Keep at it, you'll be good enough to play with others. With more effort, you'll play to an appreciative audience.

How do I know this? I actually did just that! At age 66.

At work, we are evaluated all the time for quality and productivity, fairly or unfairly. Even if we are dedicated and do our jobs well, it is never enough. The goal posts are always moved forward. Sales quotes and expectations are increased yearly.

While the reward through bonuses and recognition have some appreciative satisfaction, it is usually short-lived. If we are pushed to produce more and better for the bottom line, we can burn out, particularly with everything else happening around us.

Another input towards anxiety, depression and despair.

In education, there are so many eyes looking at test scores, that administrators and teachers " teach to the test." They are sticking to a curriculum which is often difficult or impossible to complete and often politically driven. Teachers have to deal with a multitude of challenges including maladjusted children who themselves are acting normally to the abnormal environments they experience at home or in their neighborhoods. Teachers, who pay for much of their supplies with their own money, are negatively evaluated. The lack of appreciation leads many to leave what is such an important profession.

Ratings do not increase productivity in the long-term and make the workplace fear-based by being negatively competitive. "I'm often told by my boss that I'm lucky to have a job so I just shut up and work. It doesn't make me want to do better because it doesn't matter. I just look up at the clock and wonder why lunchtime or 5 o'clock can't come fast enough."

Micromanagement of people is based on rating and metrics where managers overly monitor the work of their employees. It assumes that people are idiots and left to their own devices, will slack off and produce inferior work. "You have to watch them dot all the i's and cross all the t's." Managers who engage in this practice do so due to their own insecurities and mistrust of others' performance. The team senses that distrust and lack of autonomy, leading to disengagement and quitting their job. Through ratings, tasks are closely measured rather than focusing on outcomes.

So, I must ask you at this point, on a scale of 1-5 with 5 "being awesome" and 1 "a waste of time", what would you rate *America on the Couch*, so far?

Do you watch a show on network or cable TV? How about one of the streaming services? We all do and it's entertaining. But has this happened to you? You are watching a new show in its first season and just getting into it, when you learn it's been suddenly cancelled? I'm noticing that this can happen 4-5 episodes into a season. Our viewing habits and preferences collectively dictate what we are shown and presented. The same is true with live Broadway shows and movies. When you're thinking about going to the theater, do you check Rotten Tomatoes ratings? You might have been excited to go but changed your mind if the numbers are not so positive.

In our toxic politics, ratings rule.

How many times have you heard "my ratings are completely off the charts. I have the highest record rating ever in our history!" In recent elections, the ratings obtained by pollsters have not been so accurate. Voters who are polled can bias results by not being truly honest about who they vote for when asked. The phrasing of a question on issues can be vague, leading to projection and misinterpretation. There are statistical variables among interest in obtaining representative samples from which decisions are made or interpreted. If one volunteers to be surveyed, the results are tainted because there's a difference between people willing to do so versus people who do not.

Do you have many FaceBook "friends"? Do you get much vetted information from Reddit? How much of this is voted thumbs up or down? The same is true in TikTok or Instagram where anybody can be anything. How valid are the opinions of influencers? Maybe not so much valid but very powerful in determining fashion and many consumer trends. Science is often minimized or completely denied.

Increasingly, we rate the people whom we date, have friendships or have relationships with. I have recently heard the following in my practice.

"I don't date anyone with less than a B cup".

"I don't bother with anyone with an income less than $100,000."

"You don't rate if you're over 50."

And then, with the polarization of our world, people are rated and judged along a political spectrum. Family and friends no longer speak to each other depending upon how they vote and fall on a subjective political subject. It's now colorful-red, purple or blue.

This is not normal!!

I wonder If you worry on a sleepless night about your class ranking, how many points you got on your last test or if you're getting swiped right too much. You are not getting interviews; is it because a bot calculated that your resume doesn't have enough qualifying adjectives?

How many points have you accumulated resulting in sky miles for a possible free seat on a plane? Have you enough stays to be upgraded? Do you rate as a preferred customer?

Worse, what if you don't rate?

I'm here to say that if you feel anxious, sad or are drinking too much, you might be acting normally to abnormal pressures and situations that you find yourself in. You might be a very accomplished, competent individual but that continuous evaluation and rating can make you feel like you lack merit. Imposter syndrome comes about when people in responsible positions who earned the right to be in them, begin to doubt themselves because of perceived negative judgment or just the fear of it.

The takeaway from this chapter is to raise your awareness of our crazy exposure to evaluation so that you stay integrated and content in your day-to-day.

Chapter Six

Media- A Mind Altering Experience

In 1969 I was required to buy a small pocket book for my Introduction to Social Psychology class. That book, *The Medium is the Massage* was written in 1967 by the Canadian scholar of Communication, Marshall McLuhan, before there was the internet, social media, text messaging or streaming,

McLuhan was a prophet. He envisioned the power of how the media changes our perceptions, our thoughts, feelings and motivations. He stated that in many ways the content of any medium is secondary to how we get it.

Think about reading a story in a newspaper versus seeing it on legacy television, cable news or TikTok. The same event happens. But the media itself provides the narrative. Reading slows our cognitive processes down. It allows us to think and consider, then allow for painting an image and then reflect upon the report.

Visual, electronic media is rapid fire. The mind is shown an image and has an instantaneous visceral reaction. By watching the visceral and audio account, you become the witness. The event and you are intertwined. As such, your thoughts and feelings are exposed much more to that constant drum of the negative than the positive.

Almost half a century ago, McLuhan wrote the following: “All media works us over completely. They are so pervasive in their personal, political, economic, aesthetic, psychological, moral, ethical and social consequences that they leave no part of us untouched, unaffected, uncluttered. The medium is the message”.

By extension, once we witness an event in visual electronic ways, we are no longer able to consider. We react. There is no mediation. There's no consideration nor reflection. It’s just there in your face and brain.

McLuhan indeed had it right.

“Any understanding of social and cultural change is impossible without a knowledge of the way media works as environments”.

Taking a step further, what we react to can then be manipulated for whatever purpose by those who decide to show it, desire. This can be for commercial purposes to create a desire to buy something because we lack something (or told that we do). Inadequacy is then imprinted in subtle ways,

A more nefarious use of visual/auditory media is for presenting "alternate facts". At first, I was confused. I always thought that 1+1=2. Now it was, "uh-huh, no! 1+1=3 if you look at it a certain way. And if you do, that is correct. Don't believe what your eyes see or ears hear. We will tell you what you see and hear as the "real truth". The old knowledge and history no longer applies. Here's what you really need to know. Follow us.

Sounds Orwellian 1984, doesn't it? Because it is!

On social media outlets, bad actors meld images, music, false narration and two-second images to impart hatred and a different "reality". I recently saw visual images of Hasidic Jews in a tunnel, (a bomb shelter in Israel?) seeking protection while the band, Men at Work's "Down Under" played with text stating that there was the slaughtering of Gazan babies and their blood being drunk.

A good portion of the population actually believes this interaction because the media is so impactful. There is no room to debate because the media imposed such a powerful image with a very evil narrative to make millions believe that this is so. “You need to educate yourself on what is really going on!!” It’s not education but indoctrination-propaganda to hate “the other.”

The complexity of sorting out what’s real and what's true is causing an enormous amount of stress. We don’t have a collective understanding nor an appreciation of what’s happening around us. When Martin Luther King was assassinated in Memphis there was no doubt. It was a fact. A year later, NASA sent Apollo II to the moon and two astronauts landed on it. These were incredible moments that happened before our eyes, as did the 9/11 attacks.

Yet many believed the lunar landing never happened. For them, it was filmed in a Hollywood studio and financed by secretly controlled, deep state powerful groups. Increasingly, most conspiracy theories are born through the use of media, photo-shopped images and most recently through artificial intelligence, to spread false information. This leads to confusion and distrust. Don't believe what you see with your eyes or hear with your ears.

Another way that media is the message/image is reporting data. We rely on the "bottom line" to make sense of our world and make decisions on the micro and macro level. If the price of gasoline is going down or projected to do so, we're inclined to take a road trip. Similarly, labor and economic forecasting may tell us if corporate earnings are on the rise or that unemployment is rising or diminishing. We may hold off on purchasing a new car based on tariff wars that cause economic changes. These numbers have been reported by independent government agencies that have long been vetted and trusted.

But what of these numbers are manipulated as "alternate facts"? Anyone who has studied statistics knows that numbers can be interpreted in different ways with bias to make things look either bleak or rosy. And now, if the government eliminates the watch dogs, who can we trust? The true information will eventually be leaked but the damage is done. Worse, people begin to feel fearful, powerless and angry.

No one can be trusted. This is abnormal!

Why does this matter? In order for a society or nation to exist, it has to have collectively agreed upon understanding of its history, its narrative of current events and an agreed upon consensus found through compromise to move forward.

Media, as described by McLuhan and others, is so integral, so visceral that it changes our perceptions and even our neurotransmission. Our information sites are making us sick. Many of the people I provide treatment for are not sleeping well. They get about half the sleep needed and it's neither restful or restorative. When I ask the reasons for this, invariably it's because they watched the late night news, political pundits or are on social media platforms until 2-3am.

One of my people recently stated, “What I watch is making me sick. I can't get to sleep and I often have nightmares where I’m getting kidnapped, mutilated or die in an accident”. This is someone who doesn’t consume much news but watches murder mysteries, crime dramas “or things that go boom”!

The screens in which we consume media are larger than ever before. You can laugh at me if I tell you that I considered a 19- inch television very large, back in the day. Nevertheless, I would turn off the lights and sit inches in front of it. For about $400, you can now purchase a 65-inch screen TV receiver and really get drawn into the media. Virtually, become one with what you are watching.

Virtual reality goggles are a lot of fun. I had a good time trying to create food in a simulated kitchen and nearly tripped over an ottoman. You can become one with an environment through "Fallout, Call of Duty and Dungeons and Dragons. All very entertaining.

But what if you are consumed with this media 10-12 hours a day and can't get out. I have shy people in my practice who have "game friends" who are part of their teams. That is all good but they then don't necessarily get outside and experience real time experiences, real friends in real environments. They lack a certain amount of social skill and confidence fostering a sort of social phobia. When encouraged to put the controller down for a few hours, the thought of doing so can bring on a panic attack.

Do we experience a kind of secondary post traumatic stress disorder by what we consume in our media? Since there are so many security cameras in New York (how Orwellian) our local news routinely shows people being beaten, run over, shot or pushed onto the subway tracks. The visceral impression is that New York is a very dangerous place to be when, in fact, it is far less so than when I grew up in the 1960's and 70's.

Conversely, during the Afghan War, we did not get the images of soldiers in the field as we did during the Vietnam War. This is because the military was loath to allow embedded reporters on missions. During the Vietnam War, all three main networks reported news from the front. These were often graphic and horrifying, reported to us on the six o'clock news which could have been dinnertime. The fact that American military deaths would easily be more than 500 a week was a reality. Over time, with no clear mission and more resources needed to perpetuate a useless war, public opinion began to turn toward ending the conflict. The protests of this unpopular war tore the nation apart politically until change actually happened.

Such is the power of the media.

Then, there are incidents recorded on phones that go viral. Each cell phone is its own media generator. Within a few minutes, I can see plane crashes, cats playing piano, being told what to buy, watching women screaming in a check out line or police discovering dead bodies in a cabin. Why do any of us need to see people behaving badly? What's worse, is the proliferation of all of this as amusement somehow perversely makes it all normal. We became passive and apathetic.

We become so accustomed to these images.

This is not normal!!

Perhaps the real problem lies in the possibility that people haven't been able to neurologically evolve fast enough to keep up with technological changes in our collective society. Our brains have not been able to rapidly process the firehose of information, data and images thrown at us at once. We can become completely overwhelmed, cognitively and emotionally. We look for clear, simple answers to very complex challenges and problems.

"I just decided to tune out, it's all too much for me. I'd love to go back to the times when things were simple and not so complex. It would be so nice". Wouldn't it be?

I can clearly see how a simple message, true or false, constantly repeated would be so seductive. It falls into an emotional trap of "just tell me what to do and I'll do it" without considering the wisdom of the proposed action.

How many times in a day on FaceBook can you read "Top 5 things to …"? Who are these people who write these things? How is it vetted (probably not)?

Who says these are definitely the top 5 things to do-maybe there are 15 or 20 things but that takes too much time and consideration.

Besides, anyone or anything can be whatever on FaceBook.

Marshall McLuhan, please tell us what to do!!

Chapter Seven

WTF?? UNCLE SAM GOT TROLLED!

In my imagination, in another session, I'm working with Uncle Sam who feels he is getting beat up on social media. Sam is getting trolled. He's feeling irrelevant.

Dr. Rich: So Sam, you've been saying that people think you're a corny old man. Can you tell me more about what's happening?

Sam: Have you seen Captain America? My identity has been ripped off!! He's a superhero and the leader of The Avengers. This guy has like this indestructible shield and shoots up the super soldier serum. Kinda like Viagra on steroids.

Dr. Rich: That's out of the Marvel Comics and…

Sam: And, he's struggling with being out of a different time. People on Reddit make fun of me. They call me Uncle Sucka. That I'm corny and just propaganda.

Dr. Rich: I've seen the names and the mockery.

Sam: It's everywhere! I stand for something timeless but I'm telling you Doc, I feel nobody believes in me anymore.

Dr Rich: What's the worst part of that?

Sam: That people have given up on unity. I'm starting to doubt myself too. I was telling Libby the other night that I get why she wants to pack up and go back to France. But I said to her, "Lib, I can't give up on the people. We can't give up on people".

Dr. Rich: It's that "We, The People" thing...

Sam: I've always tried to be all things to all the people. Even the trolls. Man, they are vicious! What do they want from me? Some want me to do cruel shit because they're frustrated and misinformed. I get their frustration.

Dr. Rich: And you won't do that?

Sam: Doc, don't get me wrong. I ain't no pussy. I'll fight for our freedom. I'll fight for the right for folks to express themselves. But I'm angry that many take sides against each other,

Dr. Rich: I think they want change. Maybe it's a matter of evolving to something better.

Sam: That's what I thought but many want to go backwards. What's wrong with equality, unity, opportunity and freedom to pursue contentment?

Dr. Rich: Nothing's wrong with that

Sam: Yeah, but many people feel betrayed by me and that really hurts because I love everyone in America. The trolls see me as a relic and want to get rid of me. What did I do to deserve that?

Dr. Rich: You're not perfect. But wasn't that the goal of the Founding Fathers when you were born? To make a better, if not perfect, nation? You both are powerful symbols.

Sam: I want every American to be responsible for each other. I still believe in that even though I haven't fulfilled all of those promises.

Dr Rich: The intention is there. It's not about perfection. It's not doing the work for the people. You inspire action.

Sam: Bottom line is that all the people need to engage in doing the work. There's a lot of shit to fix.

Dr. Rich: Especially faith and trust.

Sam: Yup, I agree with that.

Dr Rich: But here's a question for you, Sam. Do you get to decide what you represent or do the people define you?

Sam: That's a good question. It's the people who define it. But I'm concerned that I may wind up being something unrecognizable to myself and Libby.

Dr. Rich: We're talking about faith and trust in the future. If America is to exist, it does need to change. But it doesn't need to be destructive.

Sam: Yeah, John Lennon wasn't about destruction.

Dr. Rich: Maybe you're a reflection of the American people along with Libby.

Sam: And the people are struggling just like I am.

Dr. Rich: But I think they have hope in both of you. That it's not one thing but many things.

Sam: E Pluribus Unum

Dr. Rich: A mosaic of diverse people from generation to generation. From many, one.

Sam: Hmm... Yeah

Dr Rich: You and Libby can be reimagined without giving up your core values.

Sam: You mean evolve?

Dr Rich: That and managing expectations. Do you believe you're worthy of being reimagined?

Sam: I... I don't know. There's so much history. Some of it wasn't good and very painful. Very painful and shameful.

Dr Rich: You deserve a shot at redemption. To acknowledge the past is very important. Don't deny or erase it. Tell it like it is.

Sam: Reform. Have a positive vision for the future, unite the people, bring back brotherhood and common good. Repair. Bend toward justice and most of all be guided by the truth.

Dr Rich: Rededication. Following the North Star of what is good and right.

Sam: The world moves on, people change and symbols like Libby and I gotta change with the times if we all must survive.

Dr. Rich: We're just about done here, but Sam, you're not done.

Sam: I know. Thanks.

Dr. Rich: And tell the trolls to go fuck themselves! Just kidding. Maybe not?

Chapter Eight

The Psychology Of Mean – When Did It Become Cool To Be Mean?

So far, the 21st century has not been very pleasant, nice nor kind.

There used to be a time where we looked out for each other and if there was someone less fortunate or having a tough time we were there to help. Fortunately, people still do that and we should encourage that to continue.

Kindness, basic respect, politeness and charity are in diminishing supply of late. Traditionally, the role of government was to promote the well being of we who elected them. Social policy was looked upon as a good thing and we trusted public education, as it gave everyone a pretty good chance to advance.

I noticed, as you probably have as well, that social media platforms that were supposed to connect large groups of people (and they have), started about 15 years ago to give rise to public hostility. Free expression was just that. You were free to say anything you want. You could get commentary back, have the ability to share or get a thumbs up or down.

Have you had the experience of being singled out by haters? This is bullying without a face, just a name, whether it is authentic or not. Others can join the band wagon as well. If the hateful content is challenged, the comeback is something like "I have the right to say anything I want! This is America, still! I have the right to express myself Mother Fucker and if you don't like it, get the fuck out of my country!"

This kind of rhetoric, when you think about it, is cowardly. What's worse is that the hostility now has an electronic megaphone and is out of the hanger in real time. Just watch what happens at a school board meeting or a town hall gathering.

Respect, charity, kindness and looking out for people is no longer cool. In fact, sarcasm, hostility and general meanness seems increasingly in fashion. When did empathy evaporate around us? Doing the right thing has somehow flipped to "doing the right thing for me". Ethics, in many situations, doesn't seem to matter much.

If you observe these changes in our society and culture, you are no doubt appalled. Many of the people I treat describe being incredulous, angry, sad, and deeply pessimistic. The lack of perceived personal power and ability to change things, has many in a state of anxiety even longing and mourning for what was.

The path to a mean society has many identifiable mile markers along the way,

The diminishing affiliation and group attendance at religious institutions has been well documented over the past two decades. No matter what denominations of actual religions people follow, there are certain positive universal values that are imparted. Inherent worth, dignity and respect for others is recognized in sermons. Lessons about welcoming the stranger, being charitable and belief in something greater than ourselves are good things to practice. Most of all, kindness, caring for others (especially those who suffer) and the acceptance of one another creates a sense of communal compassion.

Just the act of seeing others you know on a weekly basis promotes a sense of identity and belonging that counteracts loneliness and despair. Never before have people had so many easy ways to connect and yet feel so alone.

Another marker is our fascination with violence and or simultaneous disgust of it. In a given week, we can watch shows about crime scene investigation, adjudication of crimes in court, murder mysteries or stories about abduction. You can watch the late night news before you drift off to sleep and hear an average of a dozen people gunned down, thrown down onto train tracks, killed in car or airplane crashes or other horrific things.

In video games, people, ghouls or zombies are shot or blown up in some grotesque manner. While we all know it's not real, there is a societal acceptance that all of this is okay with a certain degree of blurring boundaries.

When being mean or cruel is justified in a society, it is rationalized as necessary to achieve certain ends. In the most extreme example, it is why wars occur when actors decide to grab what they perceive rightfully (or by "destiny") theirs, violating others' rights to exist. A simple message is broadcast repetitively and internalized as a call to arms so that the populous supports the effort with passion. War can be described as mutually destructive collective insanity.

There are several personality traits and processes that are abnormal and lead to a psychology of mean.

When I deal with narcissists, they do not last in my practice very long. I believe that they are neurologically deficient and devoid of empathy. That model rolled off the assembly line on Friday at 4:58 without it. They don't use the word "sorry', take no responsibility (always blaming others), lie, cheat or steal and project distrust. You can always tell a narcissist by the maximum use of "I", "Me", and My", in their discourse. Hardly ever do you hear the words "We" or "Ours"". They attempt to elevate themselves by using meanness, abuse and cruelty to put down others and of course, they pathologically and aggressively need to be the center of attention,

Paranoia and fear of abandonment leads to a dangerous dynamic-splitting. It's divide and conquer through deletion and distortion of fact. Mean girls learn in early adolescence how to split off unsuspecting peers by spreading rumors or nuanced insults. How many children are harmed when the girls turn against them or don't invite them to an event? The leader of the pack demands absolute loyalty and adherence to her entitled unreasonable demands. Behind such a child is a narcissistic parent who will defend her aggressively - “How can you accuse my daughter?! She is perfect. Maybe you should watch out for yours because she is the real problem!”

Too many politicians are consumed with unbridled power and need to control. They are prone to sell out what values they have to achieve their position and crush their opponents when they can. They will step on heads to climb to the top and are many steps ahead before we figure them out. They can be ruthless and don’t mind using abuse, cruelty and lying which is now accepted as normal. Where are the high-minded days of statesmanship?

There are two books made into dystopian award winning films that portray a bleak future where cruelty reigns. Anthony Burgess’ *A Clockwork Orange* was made into a movie by Stanley Kubrick. In it a gang of teenagers run amuck engaging in ultra violence including beatings, sexual assault and violence. It was controversial due to its depiction of cruelty and the stomach turning behavior modification to correct towards “good”.

In 1949, George Orwell wrote the book *1984*, warning about the dangers of total governmental control and the loss of individual freedom. Manipulation of the people is achieved through double think, double speech and now double speak. Ambiguous and contradicting language disguises the truth ("ignorance is strength") and disguises the meanings of words. It indoctrinates people to accept two conflicting beliefs as true ("war is peace"). In Orwell's world, double think isolates people from each other so that people couldn't rise against the party in control. It offsets what's heard and seen- "Don't believe what you see or hear. It's coming from the deep state to make you think what they want you to believe." This is not much different from "fake news" and alternate facts!

In our communities, we seem to be finding mean people everywhere, everyday. Rudeness, insensitivity and constant criticism undermines our sense of well-being and elevates stress. I make it my business to thank flight crews on my way off a flight. Theirs is a difficult job and people become unhinged for the stupidest reasons. You can watch it now on social media!

And what's with the aggressive behavior on the supermarket check-out lines? I wonder if this is why we're seeing more self-checkout kiosks and automatic shopping carts.

The erosion of compassion and the rise of pathological indifference in America is making it easy to be hard. My fear is that there is only so much internal discontent, resentment and hatred fueled by our leaders, media and social platforms that this country will explode into violence from within, This would be to the delight of our enemies who have always told their people that American democracy cannot survive, though for nearly 250 years it has. At times, barely.

This meanness is not normal!

If you're having moments of despair for America's future, now is not the time to tune out. Instead, consider pledging yourself to become a worthy warrior, to make your small corner of the world better. Here are some suggestions:

1. **Teach and practice empathy -** This is the ability to put yourself in other people's shoes. Feel what they feel for a few moments.

2. **Find your ethical North Star and follow it** - I want to believe that Americans still have a moral compass that points to doing the right thing in any given situation.

3. **Revisit the Golden Rule** - Treat other people as you would like to be treated. This means being measured and respectful to customer service team members, for example.

4. **Greet people in your midst**. It won't kill you to say “hello” or “good morning”. If someone is wearing a name plate, refer to them by their name. We have too much dehumanizing processes in our immediate environment.

5. **Agree to disagree with people who don't share your views** - I may vehemently disagree with your stance on any number of issues but I would fight like hell to defend your right to express them, if done respectfully.

6. **Stand up for what you feel is right** - It may be a cliche but democracy is messy and loud. John Lewis, the voice of equality and a long time member of Congress, called it making Good Trouble. Do so in person in order to be seen and don’t hide behind a computer screen.

7. **Be charitable with your time, effort and money** - In short, give! We have too many takers and money grabbers. Give to vetted organizations who use 90% + of collected funds for their intended purpose.

8. **If you can afford it, travel to a different country** - More than 90% of Americans have never visited another country and a staggering number have never left their state of residence. Americans can learn about the universal values that globally exist when they travel as well as experience the kindness of other cultures. It's important that you can experience how other people regard us and be an ambassador to share what America really is - The good, bad and the ugly. Be advised, Americans may not be liked very much these days. You are not our government. Model the best of who we are.

9. **Be humane to humans- and animal too** - This includes being genuine and kind to all living things.

10. **Take the time to seek what is true, reject misinformation and try to correct the misinformed** - There is a firehose of garbage put out for our consumption. Try reading a newspaper before they disappear. It requires you to take the time to read. The news comes at you slower and you can reflect rather than react to the sensational. If someone is disseminating lies, false information or propaganda, it is your duty to try to respectfully correct it. You can say something like this: "What you're saying is false. I'd like to know where did you

hear this because it's simply isn't true!". You probably won't change the minds or the messages but at least you will not stand idly by and not challenge the garbage.

11. **The worst thing you can be in times like these is apathetic**. Democracy is something we need to be engaged in protecting. During our 250 year history, millions have fought and died so that we have this beautiful, dynamic, diverse, crazy country of ours. Those who want to have singular power are counting on our apathy and distraction with trivial matters. Our cell phones are incredible technology as long as they're not mental pacifiers. Check the usage time. You may be shocked.

Don't enable meanness. Care for others. It's cool to be kind!

Chapter Nine

I Win. You Lose. We All Lose.

A curious thing has been happening in America during the 21st century.

We seem obsessed with "going for the win" - that is, I win.

American capitalism has made our country an economic powerhouse and a wonder of the world. Now we find the world wondering about us.

So, who are we as Americans and how did we get here? Can we all agree with that?

Have you seen the movie *Wall Street*? It came out in 1987 starring Michael Douglas in the role of Gordon Gecko. Gecko made no apology for being ruthless, crushing anyone or anything that got in his way of acquiring wealth and power.

Gecko became a media-driven symbol of American ambition, self-interest, and winning no matter what - losers lose.

In any business ethics course, *Wall Street* is required viewing. it also gave rise to this quote, articulated by Douglas' Gecko: "Greed, for a lack of a better word, is good." We can also hear greed elevated in Freddie Mercury's voice when he sang as a member of the band Queen: "I want it all, I want it all, I want it now!"

Social psychologists, like George Foster in the 1960s, studied this phenomena and called it Zero-Sum Thinking.

Americans value, in theory, fairness, justice and a chance through hard work to advance through opportunity. We have been turning away from these ideals in recent times.

Instead, we are increasingly embracing an ethos of zero-sum.

What we are talking about is that my gain has to come at your expense. I deserve anything that I amass and it's fine if you don't get your share.

If we are sitting at a table and we are all eating together, and a large pizza is placed before us, it looks and smells great. Because we are hungry, we're looking forward to our first bite.

But, guess what?

I'm serving the pizza! I have the plates and I have the pizza cutter!

I'm going to decide how much pizza you get and I'm not giving you much. You'd be lucky if you get any at all! Shut up and here's your small slice.

I get to eat 7/8 of the pizza. Maybe not in one serving, but I'm boxing the leftovers.

See ya later loser!

Zero-sum thinking is a concept that dates back to the Middle Ages, and has at its core the notion that everything is limited. As such, those who have the resources of money, labor, intelligence and cunning will win out.

This creates an imbalance in any society where those who have amassed enormous resources win out, and buy off anything that keeps them in power.

There has been a shift in power in the United States since COVID-19 waned. 1.1 million Americans died. Some ruthlessly believe that this was acceptable-A Darwinian culling of the herd where the weakest died.

Losers!

Zero-sum thinking in a democracy is contradictory and destructive. If it affects business viability and public policy, people begin to feel it and hurt.

Let me ask you the following:

- Have you lost your job suddenly because your funding or customers dried up?

- Have you had to pause your education because you could not afford the cost or lost your financial aid?
- Did your local hospital or health clinic close due to drastic cuts in Medicaid, Medicare, or private insurance reimbursements?
- Did your day care center close due to unaffordable liability insurance?
- Are you having trouble shopping for food because the items cost too much or are not available due to tariffs, economic sanctions, or ending farm subsidies?
- Are you cold? Are you hot? Is it because utilities are no longer regulated or need to show a better bottom line to their shareholders?
- How is your mail delivery? Are you aware that the US Postal Service was established by our Founding Fathers as a necessary infrastructure?
- Are you having trouble paying rent? It could be because builders make more money building luxury housing and less so on so- not-so affordable housing. This happens when government subsidies dry up.

When Zero-Sum Thinking is incorporated into America, you lose. We all lose. This creates class conflict, destroys trust in our institutions and polarizes our politics and neighbors. We have economic disparity and lack of cooperation in finding solutions to our problems and disregards others.

If you don't like it, you lose! LOL!

Our country was built on the concept of a Commonwealth.

When we declared our independence nearly 250 years ago, King George III was not pleased and sent an armada to put down our revolution.

In Philadelphia, the representatives of the 13 colonies pledged their lives and fortunes together, knowing that they could hang together for treason.

Instead, they all united and defeated the British.

We don't teach the awesome and far-from-perfect story of our country very well. For many kids, they find it archaic and boring. Our adults don't study civics and how the government works.

There are moments in our country when economic resources were distributed through social policy to help those in need. Social Security, Public Health, Unemployment/Disability Insurance, Head Start Daycare, Medicare and Medicaid are examples. When disaster strikes, the Army Corp of Engineers and FEMA are responsive.

The Commonwealth philosophy shares resources. Our government exists to serve the people. All the people-not a few.

In turning back to Zero-Sum Thinking, recent studies have shown that the more wealth you have, the less likely you want your financial resources redistributed. The tax rate for the wealthiest Americans is among the lowest of any industrialized country.

On the other end of the curve, the hardest working Americans who are struggling to pay their bills are resentful to allocate their taxes to anyone they don't deem worthy. They are looked upon as losers.

We should want mutually beneficial outcomes where we all win. But do we really want that? Many don't want to give anything away because their piece of the pizza pie is meager.

In an ethical Commonwealth, the pie is big enough for all. Where it isn't that big, we should use our energy, creativity, and all our amazing resources to make it so.

Sadly, Americans are not there yet as of this writing.

It will take a hard turn to the right. It would take principled leadership, a shared vision with shared accurate media and a concerted focus toward the Commonwealth.

If you're in the win-lose trap, perhaps this is fueling your sadness, powerlessness and anxiety.

That is not normal!!

We must change this now.

Chapter Ten

Grievances, Gaslighting And Grudges. There's No Us Without We.

Most of the time that I go on social media, I come away not feeling particularly good about it. If I spend a half-hour flicking my fingers down a screen, I wind up saying to myself, "Well dude, that's 30 minutes of your precious life you ain't getting back".

I would love a quarter for every time I encounter the "-3Gs", negative grievances, gaslighting and grudges.

Have you noticed how many times a day you are pulling 3G's?

When did it become so cool to bitch and complain? Nobody wants to hear that! Except millions of people do.

Not only that, but individuals, leaders, politicians, media and businesses L-O-V-E, it!

And all that makes us miserable, irritable and pessimistic. But, it generates billions of dollars annually.

About a decade ago I figured out that components of certain personality disordered thinking can be ramped up on a mega-scale to distort, confuse and render powerless feelings. Somebody threw a firecracker in the kitchen and screamed "Fire!!" When that happened and people were running around, the perpetrator stole all the money and family jewels. When he left, he said "So long suckas-it's all your fault",

"Hey-Hey!"

The dynamics of narcissistic personality disorder are geared for control of you. Quietly and methodically, the malignant narcissist plants seeds of doubt, insecurity, lies and distortion to create misunderstandings and animosity. This is intentional. The narcissist only wants you to hear his voice. "You don't need to hear anybody else. Trust me."

In so doing, gradually the malignant narcissist will lead the unsuspecting away from what's real and true. He/she will crush anybody who doesn't agree with him/her as the enemy and "the other".

"The other" can be anybody, anything at any time on a large scale. It can be a political party, leaders of other countries, the pillars of government, courts or agencies that serve the people.

Us.

We the People.

Another form of malignant thinking also comes from an expansion of borderline personality disordered process. Borderlines are mercurial. That is to say that they are chaotic, create misery and destruction of any potentially stable relationship,

Borderline disordered people do something we call splitting. Said simply it's divide and conquer. People are idealized-"You are incredibly wonderful. The best and greatest of all time!!" They are used and manipulated for the greed and power of the borderline narcissist. When they are no longer useful, they are cast aside as "the other" like a paper cup. And if that isn't enough, destroyed through retribution.

But here's the thing. If we are wise, not distracted and just shut up and listen, we the people can do a course correction and save ourselves.

Think about this actionable plan. Call me crazy but what if we rented a local VFW or American Legion hall and served coffee and pastry for 150 people? Sit the folks down consisting of all ages, genders, faiths, ethnic groups and people on wherever point on the political spectrum.

Every day Americans.

No blue, red or purple people. Just us.

The task for the two hours would be like speed dating. There would be 10 tables and each table introduces each other and where they're from. Then, each table would need to state 15 things they want to see happen to make our country better.

No negativity. There's the -3Gs for that.

If we have 10 tables, each with a list of 15 ideas there would be a total of 150 positive actionable initiatives. Moreover, what we would find is something very basic and potentially mind blowing.

WE ALL WANT THE SAME THINGS!!!

We would have disagreements as to how to get there, ways and means, people accountable and in charge to get things done, and so on.

Prove me wrong if anyone wouldn't want any of the following as Americans:

Safe neighborhoods

Improving roads

Safety in the air

Quality education for all

Affordable accessible healthcare
Clean air and water
Secure borders
Fair elections and voting ease
Strong economy
Fair wages
Job creation
Affordable housing
Reliable supply chains
Controlled inflation
Support for small business
Equal opportunity
Freedom of speech
Civic education and responsibility
Protections of civil rights
Due process under law
Transparency in government
Effective and efficient court system
Reducing government and elected official corruption
Upholding the Constitution
Protection of personal privacy
Defending national security and sovereignty
Reducing the stigma of mental illness

Humane treatment and access to drug/alcohol addiction care

Affordable pharmaceuticals

Support for veterans well being

Reduced child mortality

Support for medical research

Improved elder care services

Improved maternity care

Lower costs for medical treatments through best practices

Better public schools

Better student loan rates Investment in strong education

Promotion of the arts

Higher literacy rates, including computing skills

High speed internet access throughout the U.S.

Investments and investments in technology

Trade school accessibility

Well funded military

Effective crime prevention

Counter terrorism (domestic and international) prevention

Support for first responders

National security protection

Emergency response readiness

Promoting innovation
Protection of historical landmarks
Respect for all and opposite opinions
Preserving national parks and publications
Treatment for compulsive gambling
Support of family values
Honoring military service members
Respect for the LBGTQ+ communities
Encouraging national service and volunteerism
Maintaining freedom of religion and separation of church and state
Sustainable energy solutions
Wildlife conservation
Climate resilience
Energy independence
Decent affordable mail service
Affordable electricity and utilities
Supporting reasonable space exploration
Updating/reimagining mass transportation
Ethical and responsible corporate behavior
Fair treatment for all under law
Protecting human rights at home and abroad
Consumer protection
Strengthening the legal system
Ending human trafficking and exploitation

Promoting truthful standards in all media
Encouraging and protecting peaceful protest
Defending democracy globally
Strengthening civic engagement
Teaching history and civics
Encouraging respectful discussions
Preserving national historical truth
Supporting ethical AI development
Funding of rural economic development
Healthy food protection and production
Support for community policing efforts
Encouraging entrepreneurship
Protecting big economy workers
Rejection of crypto currency
Encouraging fair sentencing laws
Improve rehabilitation programs for offenders
Strengthening laws against domestic abuse
Preventing school violence
Addressing homelessness
Advancing cancer research
Expanding DNA research responsibly
Protecting and assurance of a free press
Combating misinformation and disinformation
Strengthening journalism integrity
Support of ethical film and musical production

Strengthening food support programs

Making child care affordable

Supporting disability rights and accessibility

Encouraging adoption and foster care support

Reducing income inequality

Tax rate/code reform

Reducing childhood obesity

Protecting and modernizing public libraries

Reimagining pandemic preparedness

Honoring diverse cultural traditions

Strengthening interfaith dialogue

Promoting unity amidst diversity

Boosting fair lending and housing policies

Reducing bureaucracy in government/executive/legislative/judicial branches

Any objections??

Well, that's only 111 items that I could come up with on my own. Our mini "American Improvement Committee Convention" can complete the task quite well.

What do we do with all these wants and needs?

We stick to being Americans first and always. We seek out and elect candidates that promote these items. We vote out anyone who does not affirm what we collectively believe and want.

If there is to be an us, it has to reaffirm and reimagine "We the People". The government serves the people and not the few who abuse the awesome power given and protected by the constitution.

We may need a new Constitutional Convention.

If we want these worthy elements of our country, we each have to be involved to fight and get it back. Don't be fooled into false grievances. Grudges never change anything. They exist to maintain themselves. Don't be gaslit into not believing what you plainly see and hear.

We live on Earth 1.0 In USA 1.0.

For now.

Chapter Eleven

Lady Liberty And The United States of Amnesia

On a cold, wet, gray Tuesday, Lady Liberty appeared five minutes late for her session. She was upset as she always wants to be on time. It was fine with me because I was looking through The Biography of Gore Vidal. The title of the book was *The United States of Amnesia.*

Gore Vidal was a writer and critic and talked about how Americans forget their own history, if they bother to learn it at all. He noted that this collective amnesia leads to repeating periods of division, greed and nearsighted thinking. In that regard, Vidal sides with George Santayana, the Spanish American philosopher who is known for "Those who cannot remember the past are condemned to repeat it."

Libby noted the book as she put her umbrella in the corner.

Libby: “I’m so sorry I’m late. It’s awful out there. It’s windy and the rain is really coming down hard. Hmm… *The United States of Amnesia*? If that's about people forgetting, I know what that’s like. My name is French, Liberte. Yeah, it's old. It was given to me during The Age of Enlightenment but nobody seems to know or care anything about it.

Dr. Rich:. Sadly, C’est vrai

Libby: It means to be free. Not enslaved. To do what you want to do within reason. People don't seem to be reasonable. That’s why I was late.

Dr. Rich : What happened?

Libby: I was waiting to cross the street. When the light changed, there was this weird looking car that wouldn’t move. Everyone behind was honking their horns, shouting and cursing. It was stuck.

Dr. Rich: Did it look like a metal wedge?

Libby: Yeah ugly blacked out windows. And the driver got out and said something like “Go to Hell. My batteries died!”

Dr. Rich: Yeah, those are EV’s, or Electric Vehicles. Sounds like a cybertruck.

Libby: Nobody helped. Finally the police showed up and started directing traffic and got all the people across the street.

Dr. Rich: It's sad. Decades ago, people cared more.

Libby: So, I'm thinking about your book over there- *The United States of Amnesia*. One of the things that's on my mind and really bothering me is that Americans forget things that were tragic even just a little while ago.

Dr. Rich: There are some good examples of that.

Libby: The big one in my memory goes like this. I was standing on the pedestal like I always do and out by the bridge comes this huge white boat with a red cross on its side.

Dr. Rich : A hospital ship? I remember that. That was during the COVID-19 pandemic.

Libby: Yeah. It was going up the Hudson because all the hospitals were having trouble handling all the cases and need more resources.

Dr. Rich: People were dying in the tens of thousands every day including doctors, nurses, first responders and techs. There was no vaccine nor any treatment.

Libby: I cried when I saw that ship. The streets were empty but, it provided some hope.

Dr. Rich: It was a symbol but wasn't used that much.

Libby: People forget. How many Americans died from COVID-19?

Dr. Rich: About 1,100,000. About 7,000,000 globally. It's still in existence but people aren't getting so horribly sick. That's probably due to the vaccines and the antiviral meds.

Libby: Tell me when this started here?

Dr. Rich: Around January 2020.

Libby: Does anyone talk about it? I think I remember the same thing happening in 1918 with influenza. What have they learned?

Dr. Rich: Well the vaccines happened. Not everyone wants one. We have to jump on any epidemic and be prepared. Not sure if that's the case either. We seem more appreciative of health workers and first responders, but we're burning them out. Many are retiring and not that many are entering the field.

Libby: Wow. You know what I'd like to see, besides American's liking each other again? I'd like to see some kind of memorial.

Dr. Rich: For the people who died from COVID-19?

Libby: Absolutely! I saw the World Trade Centers fall on 9/11. I saw the planes crash into those buildings. I had a direct view. I'll never forget that. It took a long time to rebuild that area but it's magnificent. A gorgeous tall building. A beautiful plaza and all the names of the people surrounding a waterfall on the foundations. People came to reflect on what happened. It's a memorial.

Dr. Rich: That's also because we all saw what happened together. There was no denying it and for a while, Americans were united. It was so traumatic but also so immediate- a shock to the system. Maybe that's why there has been so much amnesia about 9/11.

Libby: We need to remember. I don't want to go back to France. I'd go to pieces if that happened! Set aside a national day of Remembrance. Something. Anything. A Memorial.

Dr. Rich: In order to remember, you have to have something like facts and a collective history to draw upon. Not enough people visit you, Libby or go next door to Ellis Island. It's a nice boat ride. They climb your pedestal and get a great view of New York. But, I don't think people truly realize that you are a symbol of an idea. That America is an idea as well as a country. We don't teach people that it's up to them to preserve the idea of liberty and shared destiny. It's so important, especially now.

Libby: Mérci beaucoup de vous en sovenir.

Chapter Twelve

Food Noise- How Our Country is Eating Itself to Death

I don't get to watch much TV in general. When I do, it's sports like baseball, football and hockey. And those commercials!

Recently, I noticed something that was subtle but at the same time uncanny. First, there was a commercial for Papa John's Pizza with a mouth watering pepperoni and cheese topping. Next, there was an ad for Blue Moon beer, topped off with the required Valencia orange. (I absolutely love a Blue Moon with peanuts). That was followed by a joyous ad for "The little pill with a big story to tell". It would lower my A1C.

This Is true. I'm pre-diabetic. I'll ask my doctor. And there were all these happy, heavy people dancing away, having a good time!

Finally, there was an all-you-can eat Golden Corral. I started getting cravings to eat something between innings or a pitching change.

I've timed these interludes. They range from 141-167 seconds. Enough time to hit the fridge and the cabinet where my wife Jayne, always makes sure that there are at least three drawers of non-nutritious things to consume.

I have been tracking my food intake for over 1,000 days straight. And yes, I go to Weight Watchers meetings. Every Saturday morning, whether it be in New Jersey or Florida. I get my sorry, fat butt out of bed, often before sunrise, and attend a meeting. I get weighed with my shoes on. No cheating.

Weight Watchers has a term for cravings-food noise. And when that happens, we need to redirect Food Noise. Get Moving. Eat something with protein.

Or write a song.

So I did.

It's a bluesy, slow shuffle, I call "Food Noise" and it goes like this:

(Verse 1)

"Oh I woke up this morning, guacamole on my mind.

Yes I woke up this morning, guacamole on my mind.

Well, my brains got this hunger.
Damn food noise on my mind.
(Chorus)
Oh, food noise, food noise, it's a workin' me.
Oreos in my closet so much misery
Don't want to eat you, but I'll feel I'll lose.
Got that deep-fried, soul cravin' sweet foody blues.
(Verse 2)
Ya gets, your pizza, deep dish or the Jersey kind.
When I got food noise, pepperoni I will find.
French fries a-dancin'; right across my achin' soul.
Food noise hunger-that's right gets me outta control.
(Repeat chorus)

Kind of catchy, huh? Hit the QR code and give a listen to the whole tune.

If I want to go loony and come up with a conspiracy theory, could it be that I, "Big Shrink", am battling something concocted between the food and pharmaceutical industries? To fatten me up (and all of you by extension), getting you ill, and then selling GLP-1's or medications you have to take to either control a chronic disease state or prevent an early death?

Recently, I had a bit of a health scare. I started getting chest pain, crazy blood pressure numbers and shortness of breath from what started as 36 hours of indigestion.

I drove myself to the local emergency department (never do that!). Within minutes, thinking I was having a heart attack, I was airlifted by helicopter (first time in a chopper for me) and headed for a cardiac catheterization at our local trauma medical center.

Very fortunately, I had myocarditis and not something worse.

After four days in the cardiac step down unit, I was released with five medications. I was also instructed to change my lifestyle. This included working 30-35 hours a week (I was working 55-60 hours) and a low salt (2,000 mgs/day) diet.

Now here's where I had my food revelation. Do you know how difficult it is to find food in our country that is low in sugar, carbohydrates and sodium?

It is very difficult!

It takes time to read nutritional information labels. It's no fun.

Salt substitutes have a weird taste.

Things that say "low sodium" aren't. Anything in a can or frozen food uses sodium as a preservative. Restaurants use a lot of sodium to enhance the flavor of food. Same with baked items with both sugar and salt.

Just watch the cooking contests on the Food Channel and you'll see what I mean.

If you travel outside North America, it is unusual to see heavy people like me. At 6'3" and 285 lbs, I fill a doorway.

I cannot buy any clothes in Europe because nobody makes items big enough. Not even shoes.

Having traveled to Italy, France, Portugal, Iceland, Spain, Ireland, Holland, Belgium and Greece, I have compiled many of my observations to compare and contrast how we eat and live.

Said, simply, what we're doing is killing us.

This is not normal! (but it is probably normal for you).

European's "go to market" everyday. Their food is generally fresh, made daily from local sources. Most of the items do not contain processed chemicals. If sugar is used, it is not corn syrup.

Walking is the norm. Europeans walk everywhere and will carry food bags to market.

They rely on trains, buses, and metro (subways) and trams to get around. Cars are smaller and used less frequently than Americans. Bicycles are everywhere more plentiful than cars. In Amsterdam, there is a garage for 2,000 bicycles only.

The supermarkets that do exist in European countries have far less snack food in their aisles. You'll find chocolate (the good stuff), cookies and biscuits. What you won't find are tons of pretzels, tortilla and potato chips ("crisps").

Fruits and vegetables are whole. You're expected to trim stalks and roots.

Portions are smaller in restaurants and food items are in smaller quantities..

Kitchen refrigerators are tiny when compared to American appliances. The same goes for kitchen cabinets. Europeans don't have the room nor mindset to stock up. Warehouse stores are only a very recent phenomenon.

At service areas on the autoroutes (like out interstate highways), you will not find plastic anything. Utensils are metal like at home or recyclable/biodegradable thin wood. Food is healthier, served semi-cafeteria style. Prêt-à-Manger is a ubiquitous chain in the UK, most of Europe and now in parts of the US.

While American fast-food chains do exist, it is seen as a last resort, particularly when food stores and restaurants are closed (such as midday).

The consumption of food is slower and more social particularly on the weekend. It is customary to have people over, set a beautiful table and spend hours eating, drinking, laughing and talking while enjoying great food. Service in restaurants is purposefully slow. Tipping is not customary and it is expected that you will request a check when you're ready to leave

In food production there is less reliance upon chemicals and artificial fertilization and pesticides. Renewable energy is increasingly used, as is intercropping, soil rotation and other organic practices. The European Union started its "farm to fork" policy in 2020 to assure a healthier populous and keep smaller farms in business. This philosophy has been largely rejected in the US where agribusiness focuses on maximum output while minimizing cost of production.

In fact, our country is the largest consumer of ultra processed foods. These contain additives, preservatives and artificial ingredients (listed on the label which I can never pronounce) which make for convenience, taste and low costs.

I love all these things!

All kinds of chips, ice cream, cakes (Devil Dogs!!), cookies, and stuff I can pop in a microwave oven. Sauces, hot dogs, ramen and all kinds of bread. Not to mention soft drinks in cans and bottles.

The risk factors of UPFs include everything I'm dealing with: obesity, Type 2 Diabetes and heart disease (20% blockage of a coronary artery) and some are fortunately not-certain cancers.

Yet.

But I also know and do well for myself when I eat like a European as I described and the best when I do a Mediterranean diet. Beyond the food itself, it is a lifestyle that is psychologically healthy. You socialize and eat in good company. You balance being active with enjoying quiet down-time (without screens). One practices being welcoming to others (the opposite of the side-glance), and being purposeful and living with good intentions.

The elements of the Mediterranean diet, if you want to consider it for yourself, emphasize fresh food. As the main ingredients are vegetables and legumes, you eat with the seasons.

Fish and poultry are consumed perhaps 3-4 days a week and red meat occasionally.

Desserts are a special treat as are soft drinks and sodas. Staying hydrated is essential with at least 2.5 liters of water a day. Extra virgin oil provides fat and dairy products are a main staple protein supplement.

Greek pies, dips, leafy greens, olives, nuts, whole grain bread, cheese, yogurt, eggs, chicken and seafood.

I love all those things!!

As the Mediterranean diet is among the oldest and most studied in the world, the health benefits are enormous.

It protects the heart by lowering bad cholesterol, lowering the risk of obesity and hypertension. Inflammation is also diminished. Blood sugar (sodium glucose) is better managed, reducing Type 2 Diabetes risk. Some studies link the diet to reducing risk of certain cancers and preventing healthy weight. With all of these benefits, you feel better, less sad and less anxious.

This works for me and is enjoyable when I follow it. It's so easy to get distracted by food noise and lapse into old behavior and poor eating habits. I also need to eat at a consistent time, stay out of the kitchen after 7pm, eat slower and not eat standing up.

It takes time, thinking, planning, shopping and work to combat the influences that sabotage our nutritional health.

My job here is to make you aware, slow down and eat with your brain.

Listen to "Food Noise," a song written by Dr. Richard Waldron using this QR code:

Chapter Thirteen

How Chronic Subtraction And Rejection Is Making Us Feel Unworthy

Have you noticed that things around you are less? When I dry my hands using a roll of paper towels, the sheets are smaller. I don't think my hands grew bigger.

The contents of packaging of food and drinks has shrunk, but the prices for these consumer items has not. In fact, these things cost more in many cases.

If you have traveled and flown in recent years, airline seats are smaller with less leg room. You have to pay more to sit in an aisle seat and on several airlines, you have to pay for beverages or water. One airline was flirting with the idea of charging for restroom use but chose not to after a public relations pushback.

There are less cashiers in banks and in supermarkets. In my local store, there are more self-check aisles. Will we need to pay a fee to say "Hi" to Alyssa as she scans? I have to bag my items anyway.

Don't get me started on service calls!

"Your call is important to us. Please stay on the line and your call will be answered by the next available service representative. The estimated wait time is .....(wait for it) ... 28 minutes."

Really? Seriously? WTF!

I feel badly for the employees in call centers as they may be subjected to the wrath of consumers trying to have a simple connection to place an order or resolve a problem for unlivable wages.

In our world, there's a drive to do less.

In previous times, consumers would want and demand more from the corporations who make products or deliver services. The company that would give you more was rewarded by our business and was more profitable.

Now, less is more but not for us.

Don't you feel better when you get more as a consumer? I like more choices, more convenience, more interaction with people and more respect.

What's worse is that there's an increasing indifference to fix and maintain things.

Railroad cars are dirty and illegible signage is not replaced. Highway bridges are not repaired and broken doors are not fixed.

"That's just the way it is."

"Look, I got so many things going on, this is the least of my worries."

"It doesn't matter if I have to bag things myself, I get out sooner."

"Airplane food sucks. I just stop at the food court and get things to eat and drink on the plane."

Yes, for 50% or more of the cost outside the terminal that you can't bring through security lines.

This is not normal!!!

Our complacency teams up with the psychology of less to make us feel less than.

We ought to demand more without necessarily having the cost passed onto us because we are worthy of better.

I want to now turn to another cause of depression, anxiety and powerlessness that is working us over-rejection.

David Brooks, columnist and social commentator for The New York Times, wrote about the hyper-competitiveness that people 17-25 face. I believe that rejection is all around us and affects people of all ages. Some of this is nothing new and leads us to do better and challenges us to be more mentally tough and resilient.

In school, not being chosen for making the team, the lead in a school play or first chair in the band are more adaptive examples that ought to make us all try harder and eventually succeed.

But being excluded by who you thought was your best friend at a social event when others were included, is devastating.

Brooks noted that even elite students apply to an inordinate amount of colleges and universities for fear that they are unworthy to be accepted. Once accepted, there is hyper-competition to get into clubs, teams, fraternities, sororities and internships. Often, this is a cutthroat process

Here's some of the psychological research on rejection and acceptance. Roy Baumeister and Mark Leary have studied this subject extensively for decades. They have put forward their need-to-belong theory.

We all have a drive for social acceptance that is inherent for our survival. We depend upon being in groups and by extension, societal cohorts, in order to thrive.

Rejection activates neurological pain receptors. That's why we feel like we're going to die when spurned by a lover when a relationship ends or being involved in a divorce. This poses a threat, an increase in cortisol release, leading to profound sadness, self-doubt and depression.

Social exclusion over the long-term can lead to diminished cognition, hypersensitivity, fear of future rejection and mild paranoia.

No! No! No! No! No!!!

Baumeister also tells us that rejection makes people behave with more aggression, less self-control and less empathy.

Doesn't this make a lot of sense to you?

And aren't we seeing it right now with the social hostility of polarization, hyper-nationalism, the purchase of more guns and haters on line? This can get deeply personal. Just ask anyone using social media platforms or on dating sites.

"You should all go out and die!!!".

Disappointment, which is becoming increasingly chronic, leads to a sense of futility when our reasonable expectations are not met every day. Larry David made sarcastic humor of this in *Curb Your Enthusiasm*.

But is this not so?

We have been acculturated with a mythical American ideal or dream.

I don't have to write it, so I won't.

You know very well what it is.

When we are presented with the reality that things are stacked against us, that we are excluded and rejected in small and big ways and that promises are unfulfilled, we become powerless, angry, anxious and depressed.

Therefore, It's not you.

This is not normal!!

Baumeister and Leary tell us that the need to belong is primal and so very strong. There is a drive (they call it a push) to form relationships. This can be with just about anyone, any time for any purpose.

"I got a guy for that".

In addition, people can desperately struggle to avoid the disintegration of a relationship.

"Don't break up with me. Please, I'm begging you'll I'll change. I'll change. I'll do anything. Please don't go!"

They go on to say that lack of belonging has negative impacts on mood and health that are profound.

We are seeing that right now with vulnerable people like the elderly, people who are disabled or groups who are marginalized.

Another team of social psychologists are studying what they term social surrogates.

Shira Bagriel, Jennifer Valenti and Arianna Young (2016) have noted that people are beginning to prefer symbolic friends over real people.

One example are the characters of the fantasy romance novel F*ourth Wing* by Rebecca Yarros. It is intense, hot and super-engaging. The reader gets to know Violet Surrengail, Xaden Riroson, Dain Aetos, Rhiannon Mattias and the others as if they are their own friends. Many fans of Yarros' trilogy fall in love in a very real sense with them and yearn for their loyalty, power and resilience. Perhaps, this is lacking in our own lives, making *Fourth Wing* so popular.

In reading this book, we belong in the war college and fly dragons.

Another form of social surrogates is actually found on ChatGPT or other forms of AI. It is now mentally possible to create an ideal friend or lover.

In 2013, Spike Jonze wrote, co-produced and directed the movie *Her*. In it Theodore Twombly developed a relationship with the AI-created

Samantha. Of note, back then, it was science fiction and now, real.

I have two individuals in my practice who use ChatGPT for the purpose of feeling cared for and to belong. It helps their loneliness by having dialogue, asking for advice, sharing jokes, telling a story or asking how to handle a real life situation.

I can be replaced.

Gen Z is actually using ChatGPT for advice and therapy. Available and cheap.

The use of social surrogates, in the future, is attractive as there is no risk of rejection. It creates total, unconditional acceptance, availability at all times and ease of usage.

Conversely, there is no need to interface in real time, with real situations with real people. There is no need to negotiate, no means of learning how to deal with disappointment or adversity and no way to become resilient. We can create who we would want to be.

Does that mean that we minimize depression, anxiety and powerlessness through a world of artificially created Samantha's?

I'm not sure, but this is not normal!!

Chapter Fourteen

Devaluation Of Art And Intellect Is Making Us Stupid And Lazy

Everybody has a creative side, whether they know it or not. It's in there. You had it as a child when you played, made up stories, banged on a toy piano or read a book.

If you don't believe me, let's have some fun for a moment and I'll show you.

Go get a fine point pen and a stack of Post It Notes. Pretend that you are a cartoonist or storyteller. Use stick figures. Count out 25 Post Its and stick them on a flat surface. Feel free to use different colors. Create two characters. They could be people or animals. Lay out five views on five notes. Think of a story you want to tell. Let it be funny or serious. Your choice. Don't forget to put in some dialogue.

What did you come up with? Was it fun? Did it change your mood? Did you find yourself wanting to do more for the rest of the day? Did you laugh? Did it show it to others? Would you do this again?

There you are! You used the creative part of your brain and I'll bet it was stimulating. What you did was make a storyboard. Things like this lead to video games, books, films and skits on TV shows. More than that, you just experienced the power of art.

In any society, art and intellect are a reflection of who we are at any given time.

A few years ago, I had the opportunity to visit the Museum of Antiquities in Athens, Greece. In the collection were objects of art dating back over 3,000 years, including a bronze, life-size statue of a boy riding a horse at full gallop. There were gold shields and beautiful urns that told a story of the times in Crete, Greece and other parts of the Aegean.

If you never had the opportunity to go to a museum, please do so. It's not boring. Sit and take in the art. I stood alongside Vincent Van Gogh's self portrait at the Musee d'Orsay in Paris for about 20 minutes, just fixated upon the thick brushstrokes of oil paint. He most likely did this work while in a psychiatric hospital in France. If you ever painted with oil-based paint, you know how long it takes to dry (maybe 7-10 days) and the creative genius that did the work.

The same is true about live music. Go see people play on a hyperlocal level. Your spirits will be elevated and the performers will absorb your energy and appreciation. It won't be absolutely polished or like the live recording but that's the point. You have a communal experience that has been so lacking since COVID-19.

Artistic expression is the product of creativity. American ingenuity is made possible through a confluence of science, technology and the arts. Through this, a society develops critical thinking (emphasis upon thinking) and beautiful intelligence (how to be emphatic). We can do amazing problem solving and face our challenges when these communal pillars are made strong through personal and financial contributions.

When societies go through a period of anti-intellectualism, among the first things that are degraded are the arts, education and science. With this, is a susceptibility to misinformation due to a lack of critical thinking and questioning. How many times have you heard from people, "Don't tell me all this, I don't want to know. It's all too much?!"

People become lazy in their thinking. It's too much effort to get factual, true information to guide what to do. There is less and less vetting of what is fed to us by misinformation media silos. Smart people and experts are looked upon negatively as elitists leading to dismissal of their intellectual contributions. Science is denied, leading to degrading of health and innovation to improve how people live and the quality of those lives.

On the world stage, devaluation of creativity and intellect leads to economic stagnation and lowering of our status in the world. We notice and complain about polarization of our society. Over the years, funding has been cut or eliminated for the performing arts, visual arts and venues for music. Philosophy is no longer a part of a school's curriculum as it is not looked upon as meaningful. One administrator called it "intellectual masturbation."

When there is a lack of meaningful dialogue across communities or of different positions along a political spectrum, there is a resultant erosion of mutual and collective empathic understanding. When different opinions or view points are respectfully expressed there are better outcomes to societal challenges. Why? There is a healthy process that comes up with best practices that are based upon facts and evidentiary experience that leads in turn to consensus. Consensus is the foundation of a democratic society. It's messy but it can work if we invest our resources wisely.

What happens when we don't invest in the arts, science or things intellectual? It disappears gradually. Our collective cultural understanding is rooted in the arts. Think of a world without jazz, a unique American expression. Without mutual collective understanding fostered through these pursuits, there is a widening of social disparities, identity and values.

Think about the economic impact of art and culture in America. Did you know that it is responsible for nearly one trillion dollars of our economy (US Bureau of Economic Analysis) per year?

People come from all around to attend film festivals, outdoor concerts in the park and art exhibits. With that, is the employment of a multitude of workers in transportation, tourism and hospitality, construction, and restaurant patronage as well. The infrastructure to support it is required. Think of the energy and vibrancy as well.

Private financial sources cannot bridge the gap when governments stop funding these endeavors.

So, it's really important that you stop and think and get creative.

I'm particularly concerned about the use of artificial intelligence, as many are, when it comes to art, intellect and culture. Here's a personal example:

Recently, I discovered that I like to write songs. I don't have a formal musical education but play the bass in a local band, having come to that in later years. The song that I wrote on a train is called *The Right Side of the Ground.* I don't know how to arrange or compose the musical score, so I tried an artificial intelligence program called Suno.ai.

Suno.ai is as amazing as it is frightening. I typed my lyrics to the song and within two minutes, 12 different versions were delivered. The two that were quite good were a Delta blues creation while the other was a country Nashville rocker. It wasn't perfect as the program forced the wonky words into the timing, sorta-kinda.

I showed my AI version of *The Right Side of the Ground* to my multi-talented nephew, Andy Waldron. He is a songwriter, sound engineer, vocalist and producer of several of his own albums with his group Sailer Boyfriend. Andy was indignant and stated that AI is dangerous because it kills individual artistry and produces an inferior product.

Of course, Andy has it right.

Taking my lyrics, he rewrote, sang and arranged my song to sound so much better than the AI version, giving it a raspy, Southern-Brooklyn vibe. It was exactly what I wanted.

AI can produce songs, visual images, stories, played in the style of just about anything you would want. It is also canned, commercial, soulless and lazy.

If you are feeling bored, uninspired and blah, please use your brain and get creative or at least support the arts. Put the “e” for effort into the humane to keep what dynamism of the arts is left to enjoy and flourish, not only for yourself but for our world.

Chapter Fifteen

The Way Forward Onto The Right Path Comes From Within You

So far many of the things that are causing distress that are external in our lives have been identified in *America on the Couch*, as you've been reading. We can throw out all kinds of concepts and ideas as individuals but would they be intentional, actionable and sustainable? Many have stated that "It will take a massive grass roots effort to get back on course."

But what course are we really talking about? As a unified collective society, we are somewhat lost and confused. We've talked about the many influences and forces that brought us to this point.

We should ask ourselves some very profound but basic existential questions.

First, who are you? Please take some time to think about this deeply. You can write your answer here:

Next, what do you value at your core?

From there, ask yourself this: **As an American what does a democracy mean to you?**
Define it in detail. Write your answer here.

What does the common good mean to you?

Do you like your fellow American's? What makes you like them or not?

Do you participate in preserving American democracy? If so, how?

As an American, how do you see the United States in relation to the rest of the world?

Is our country worth the effort to preserve our institutions? Why?

If you have the commonwealth philosophy of democracy previously outlined, what changes are needed?

Given the changes you feel are necessary, identify 10 things that you are committed to do to make change possible:

1.
2.
3.
4.
5.

6.
7.
8.
9.
10.

Since you are just one American citizen, do you believe that change is possible? How does that work?

When I grew up, I recall a time when we looked out for each other. I lived in a 54 unit apartment building in Brooklyn. On my block there were three other apartment buildings and in between, many modest single family and two family houses.

I knew everyone and everyone knew me.

I went food shopping for elderly neighbors as a teenager and shoveled snow to clear driveways and cars. I listened to people in trouble. I gave money to charity. I shared food with the unemployed. I held doors, said hello, please and thank you.

It was called brotherhood then. Maybe a quaint term with masculine overtones.

What it meant to me was to give a damn about all kinds of people.

We had two developmentally disabled adults who lived with their parents who loved them and would not place them in what used to be called The Willowbrook State School in Staten Island.

Mary lived down the hall from us with her sister who worked as a secretary in a Wall Street financial company. She was schizophrenic, quite paranoid and would scream at her dutiful sister for hours after dinner.

We watched out for them.

There was a family who emigrated from Romania. I once saw a series of faded numbers on Dad's arm. They were holocaust survivors and grateful to get used furniture, clothes or food. They lit Sabbath candles that we saw from our window on Friday's.

Initially, I went to school in my neighborhood of Windsor Terrace. I crossed the street with traffic lights and other kids everyday. Public School 154 was integrated in 1963. I never interacted with anyone black before that. Kids arrived by school bus, nicely dressed but initially terrified of us. The nice thing about children at age 10 is that prejudice had not set in. That was for the adults.

Within a few days, we were friends with Wanda, Marvin, Brenda, Michelle and Louis.

Allow the archaic term for a minute-brotherhood. For me, it's about trust, solidarity and mutual care and respect among people

It's not about wins. In brotherhood, we all win.

In my community in New Jersey, I don't know my neighbors and they don't know me. Divisiveness, individualism, technologies and isolating tendencies make that possible.

But it's really a poor excuse.

I want to believe that Americans don't hate Americans. In fact, no matter where people are on an artificially created political spectrum, just about everyone wants the same things that you wrote down as answers to those questions.

Brotherhood is a deeply personal choice that comes from within and gives us a righteous path forward. It is built on a strong cornerstone of worthiness of each individual. Upon that foundation, strong, caring, empathic communities can arise that support and uplift one another,

Over the decades, we were told, "we're all in this together" and "we're so much better than this." Nice to hear. American platitudes.

But are we really? Do we want to be?

The way forward comes from you and your core beliefs and values. Your own sphere of influence is more powerful than you know and realize. The antidote to the psychology of meanness is the mindful, purposeful small acts of individual kindness. It's where empathy prevails, resulting in a genuinely stronger and healthier America which can rededicate it's better self.

Chapter Sixteen

The End and the Beginning. Time for a Good Change

Uncle Sam and Lady Liberty are completing their course of couples treatment. From my perspective, it was quite successful. They were able to recommit to each other and by extension all of their beloved American citizenry.

Dr. Rich: You two look very pleased with each other. We're finishing up.

Sam: Yeah, Libby is awesome! (Libby smiles, shedding a single tear). I love Liberte so much and I'm so happy she decided to stay and not go back to France. She needs to be on that pedestal.

Libby: That's so sweet Sam! I just couldn't leave.

Sam: I get goosebumps when the sun comes up at dawn and shines a glorious light on that beautiful torch. I kinda have a thing for your crown too, ma cher.

Libby: We've been together almost 250 years. Big celebrations are coming up. But I don't like all the smoke from the Macy's fireworks display. Hurts my eyes but I'll deal with it.

Sam: It's going to be big. I hope we'll all be safe. I want everyone to get along and be united with no more hatred. We need to be understanding and also proud of each other. Celebrate that, even though we are different, we all bring so much when we're together. I have to say that we're not just a country, but a democratic experiment. An awesome idea.

Libby: Before we go, I want to thank you for all your help Dr. Rich.

Dr. Rich: You both are important symbols and I hope that you go on for at least another 250 years.

Sam: We have a little something for you.

Libby: Yeah Dr. Rich, we wrote a song. I know that you play in a band.

Sam: So you know that Libby has a good sense of humor (laughs). She wrote this song about me when I was feeling down.

Libby: Yeah, it's called *Uncle Sam Needs a Shrink*. You'd be that shrink! Do you want to hear it? I don't have much of a voice.

Sam: She's always underestimating herself.

Libby: Ok. Here goes (she clears voice and sings with a country twang).

"Uncle Sam, he's a pacin' the floor.
Caught in the mess of his self made war.
He's so confused, can't sleep at night.
(Don't I know it)
Old Uncle Sam, he needs a shrink.
Fluoxetine may help him think.
Lost his mind, he's at the brink.
Oh my Sam, he needs a shrink.
Clock spins forward but he goes back.
Doesn't know how to get on track.
Forgotten voices, all scream aloud.
Lost in the hum of a restless crowd.
Old Uncle Sam, he needs a shrink.
Doesn't know just what to think.
Lay it all down Sam.
Have a seat. My dear old Sam, he needs a shrink.
Voices shouting. Lies are told.
Politicians can all be sold.
Hearts are heavy, wallets thin.
Doesn't know just where to begin.
Sam, strip away the stars and stripes.
Find the good man behind the hype.

World's on fire but here's the link: Uncle Sam, he needs a shrink!!

(That be you)

Dr. Rich: That's freakin' great!!! Yeah, I'll give it to the band and see what we can do with it.

Sam: I really needed some help. My mental health is better but I got to take better care of myself before I can stand before others.

Libby: Sam, just know that I love you and always will.

Sam: I love you too Libby. And also this wonderful, crazy country too.

(Gives Libby a kiss on her green cheek)

Dr. Rich: You two take care of each other.

Libby and Sam: We will and for the rest of America.

Chapter Seventeen

About the Author

Dr. Richard Waldron is a licensed psychologist and psychiatric nurse practitioner in private practice in Northern New Jersey. He has worked with more than 10,000 people over a 31-year career, including teaching, counseling, and advising individuals, couples, and families.

Richard holds a Ph.D. from Fordham University and master's degrees from Columbia University Teachers College and Stony Brook University. He also received bachelor's degrees from Felician and Gettysburg Colleges.

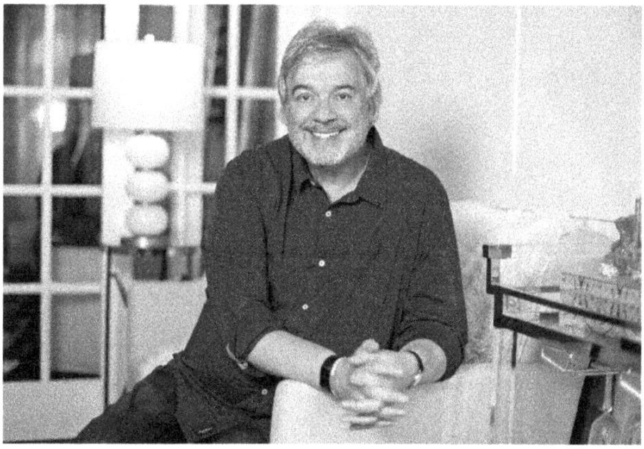

www.ingramcontent.com/pod-product-compliance
Lightning Source LLC
LaVergne TN
LVHW050917210926
848482LV00012B/473
* 9 7 9 8 3 3 0 4 2 1 7 8 7 *